The Angel Baby

Written by Katherine Craddock
Illustrated by Katie Craddock

One day, Katie's Aunt Jackie came over
to her house and told her the best news ever!

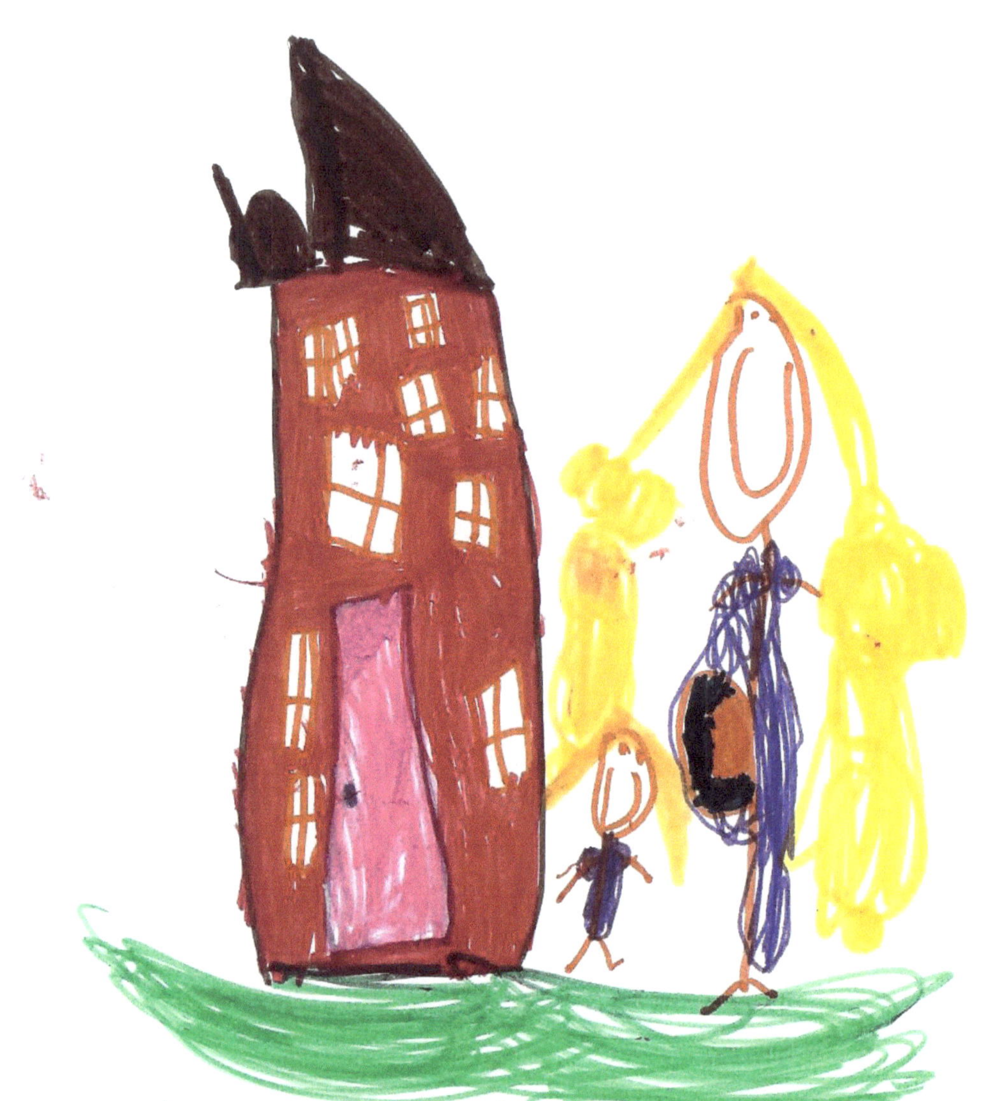

"Guess what, Katie?" her Aunt Jackie
said. "I have a baby in my tummy!"

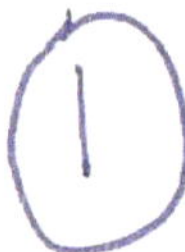

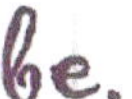

Aunt Jackie's smile was as big as could be.

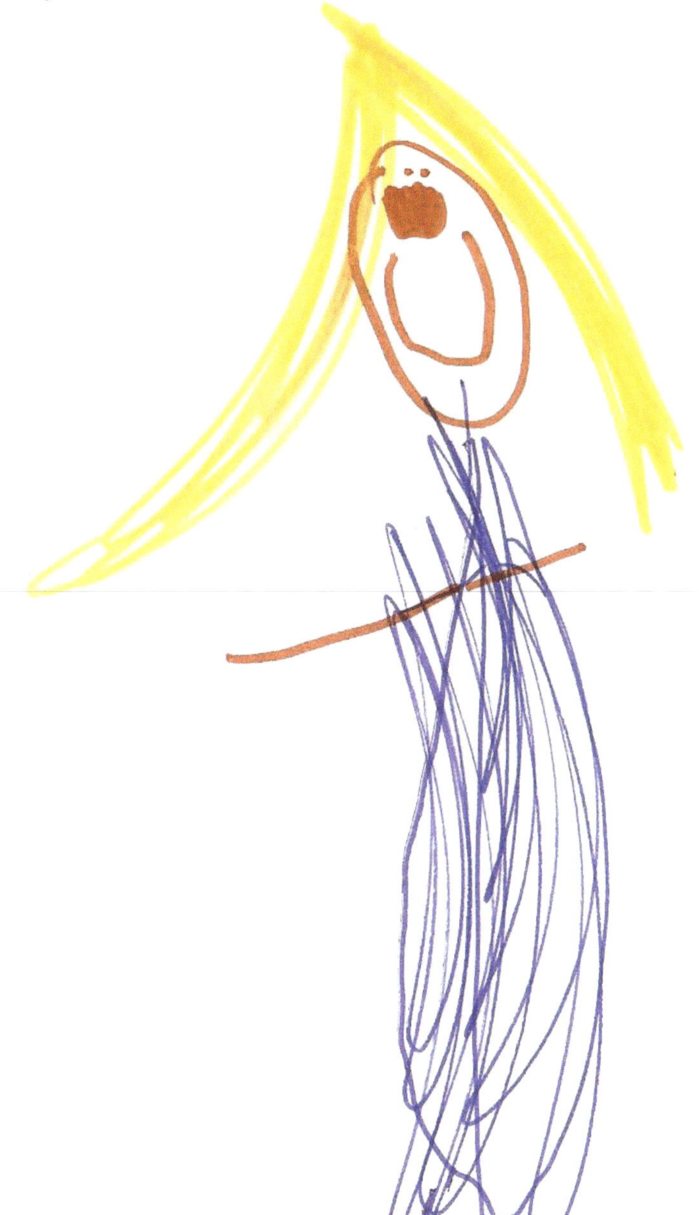

"Can I see the baby in your tummy?" Katie asked. "Right now?"

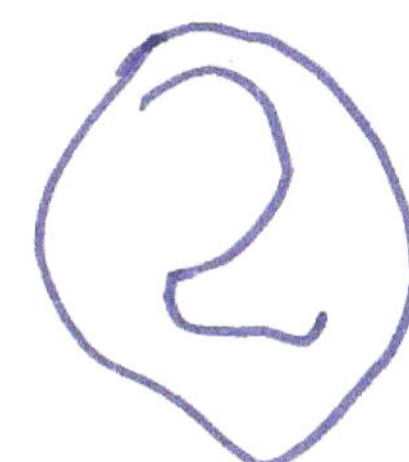

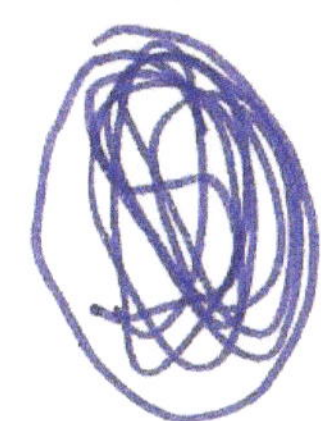

Katie was so excited! Even though the baby hadn't been born yet, she already knew all of the ways they could play together.

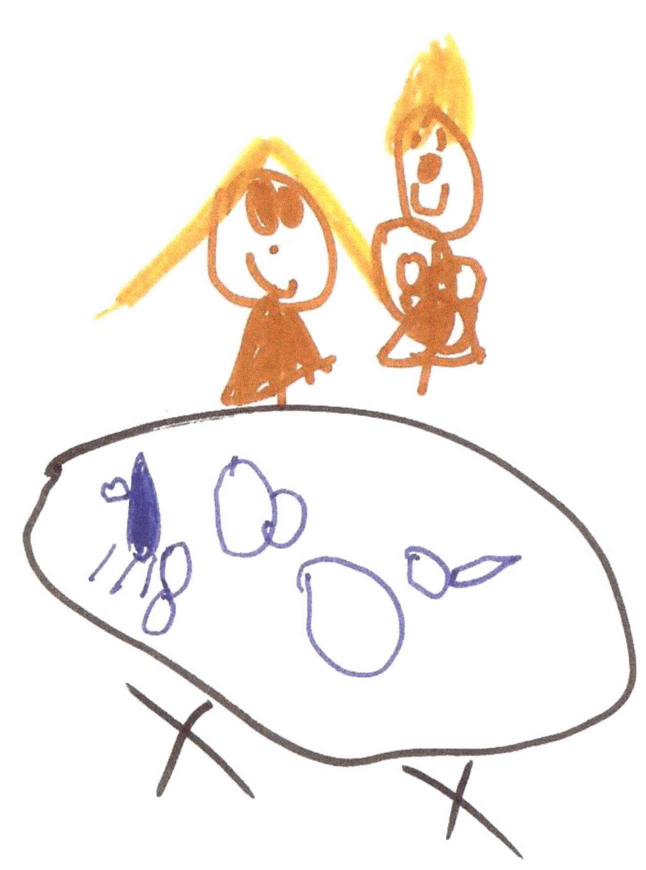

"We can have tea parties, and I can hold it, and rock it, and sing to it ..."

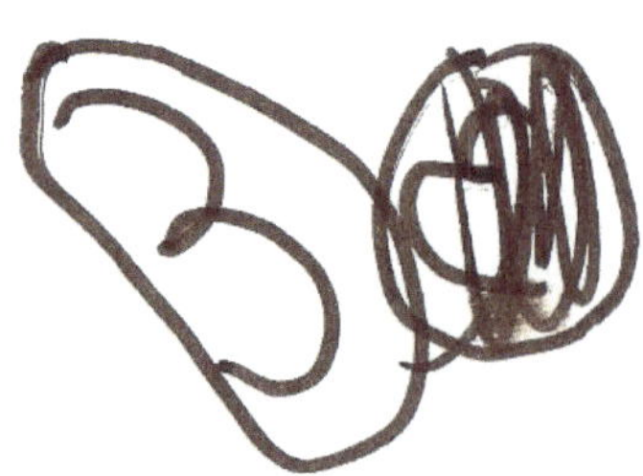

Aunt Jackie shook her head.

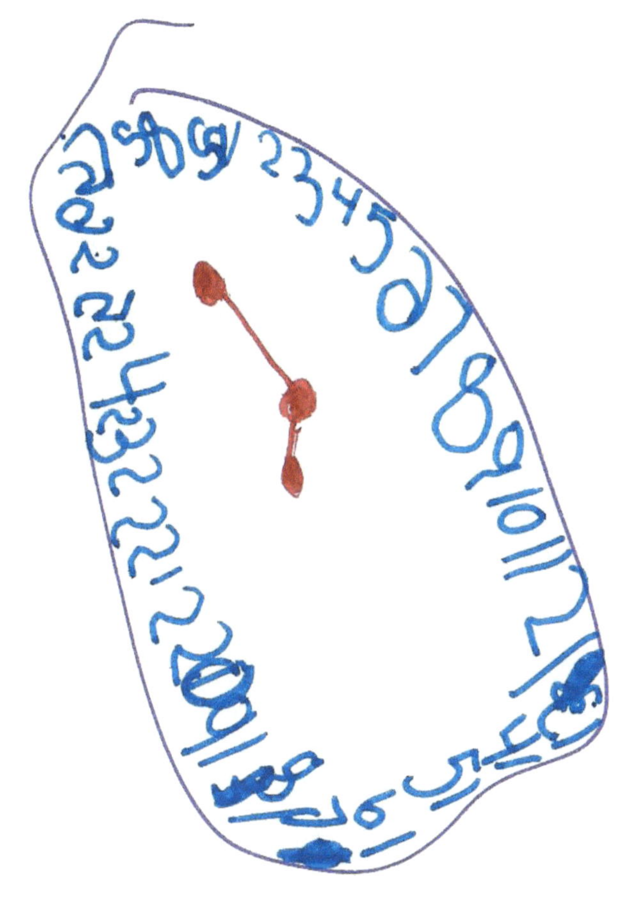

"Oh, no, Katie ... you have to wait a long time before you can see the baby. But after you wait a long, long time, THEN you can play!"

For the next few days, Katie told
everyone about the new baby that was coming.

She was _sooo_ happy, she danced and sang.

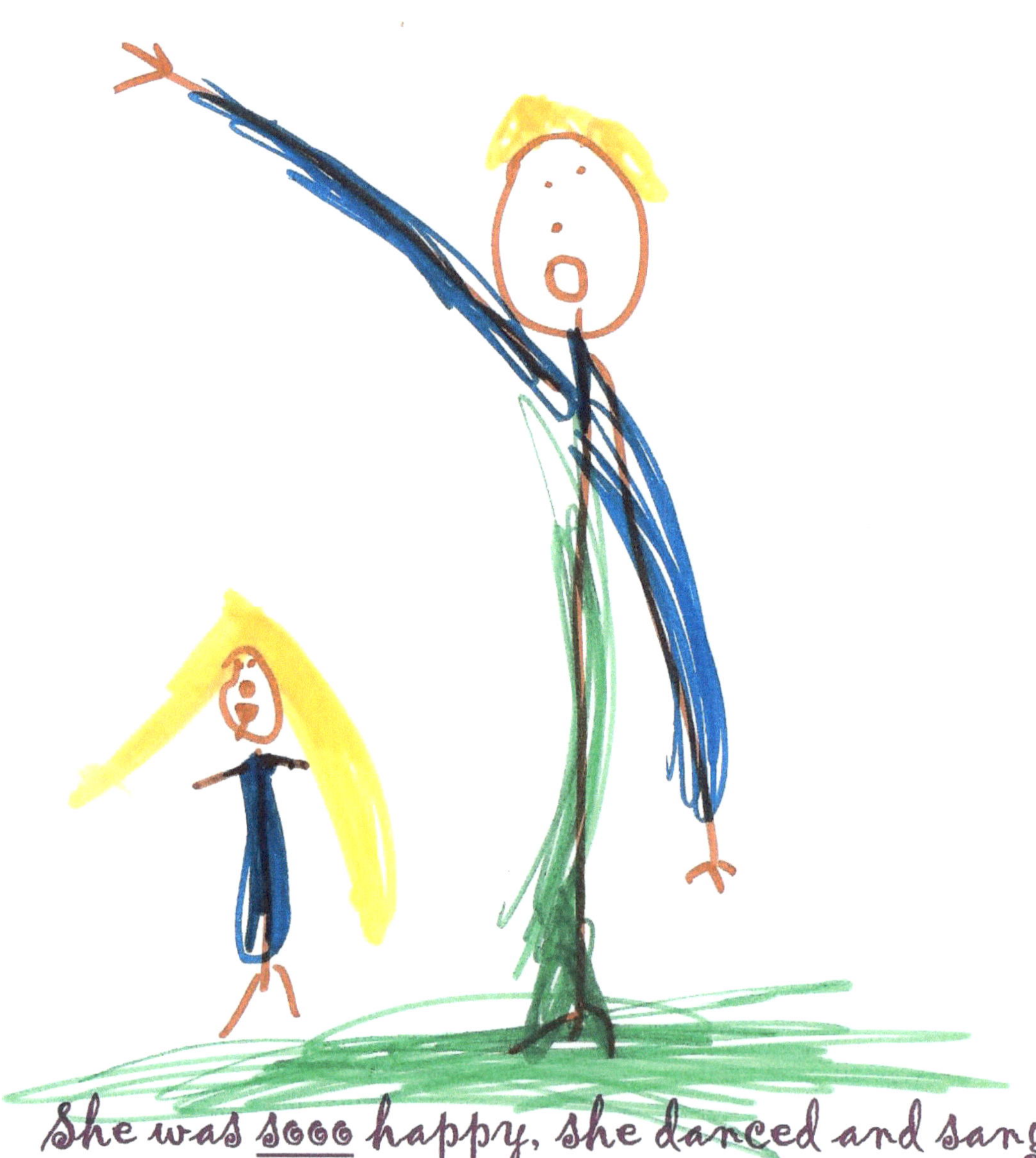

5

But the next time she saw Aunt Jackie,
Aunt Jackie had a very sad look on her face.

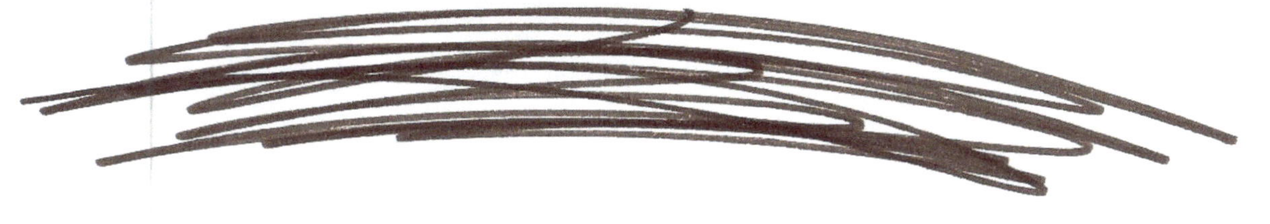

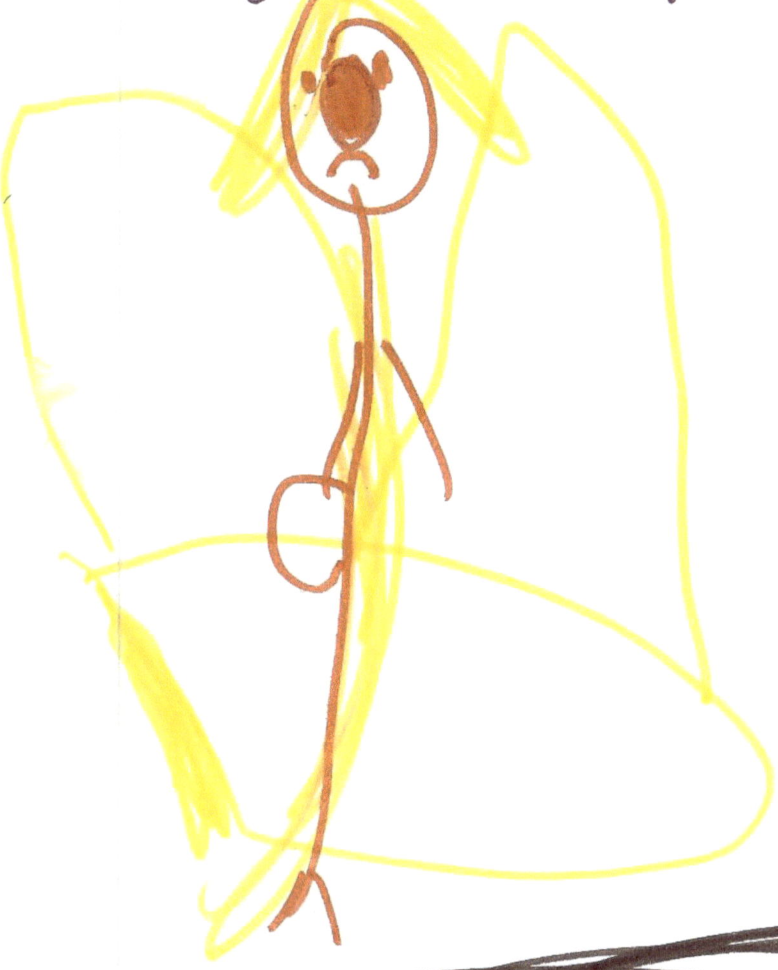

"Hello, baby!" Katie said to Aunt
Jackie's tummy. But Aunt Jackie just looked
even sadder.

6

Suddenly, Katie noticed that Aunt Jackie had a lot of funny bracelets on her arm.

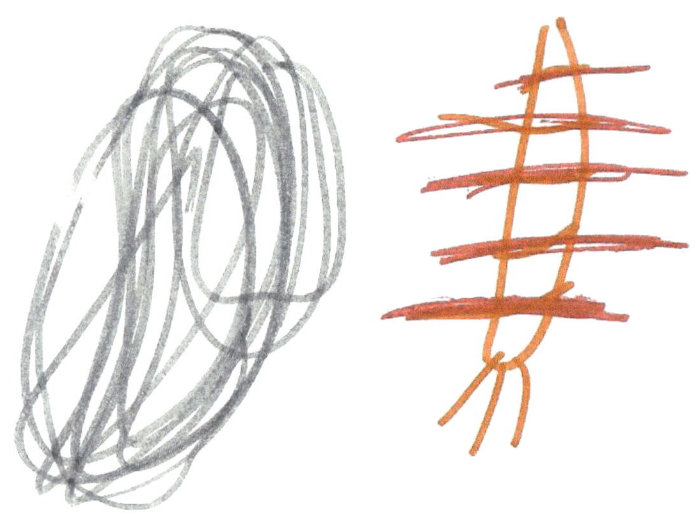

"Why do you have those bracelets on your arm?" she asked.

7

Aunt Jackie got very quiet. "I had to go to the hospital today," she said.

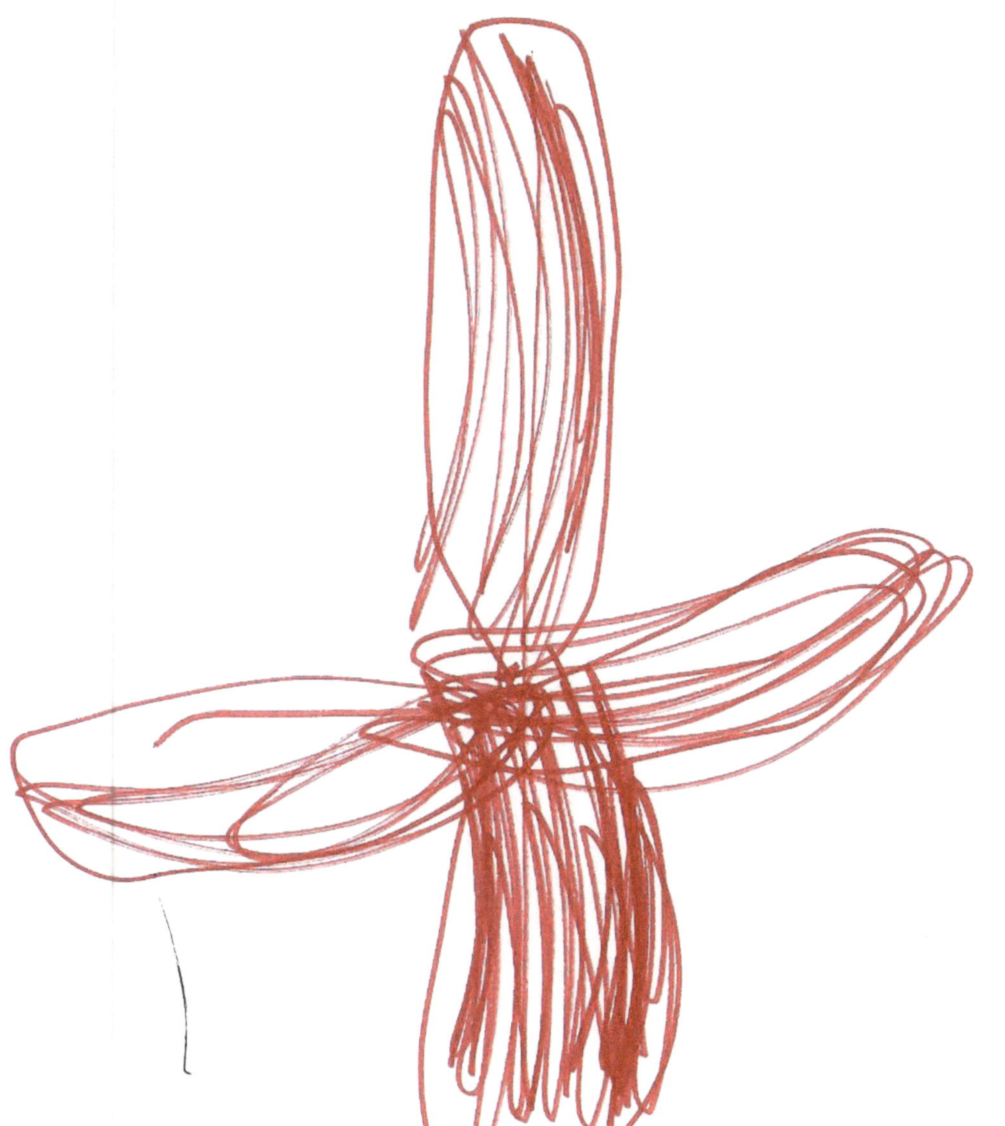

"I wasn't feeling very well. Will you say a prayer for me?"

8

Katie cuddled up in Aunt Jackie's lap
and held her tight.

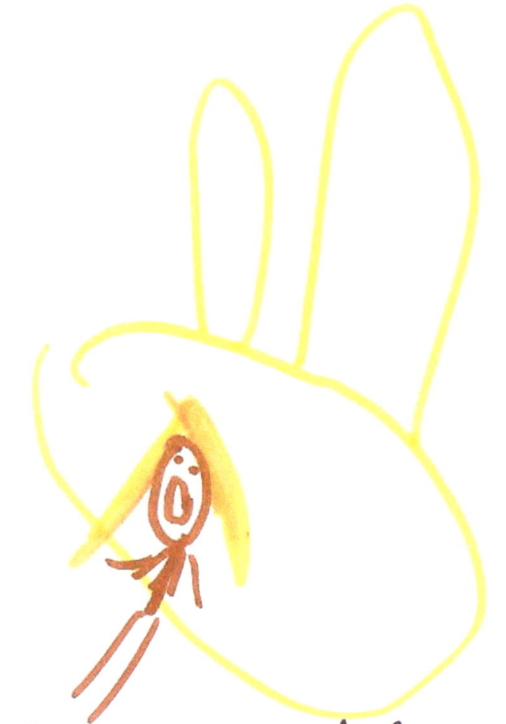

"Dear Jesus, help Aunt Jackie feel
better. And help the baby in her tummy to
feel better, too."

9

That night, Katie was worried. Why was
Aunt Jackie so sad?

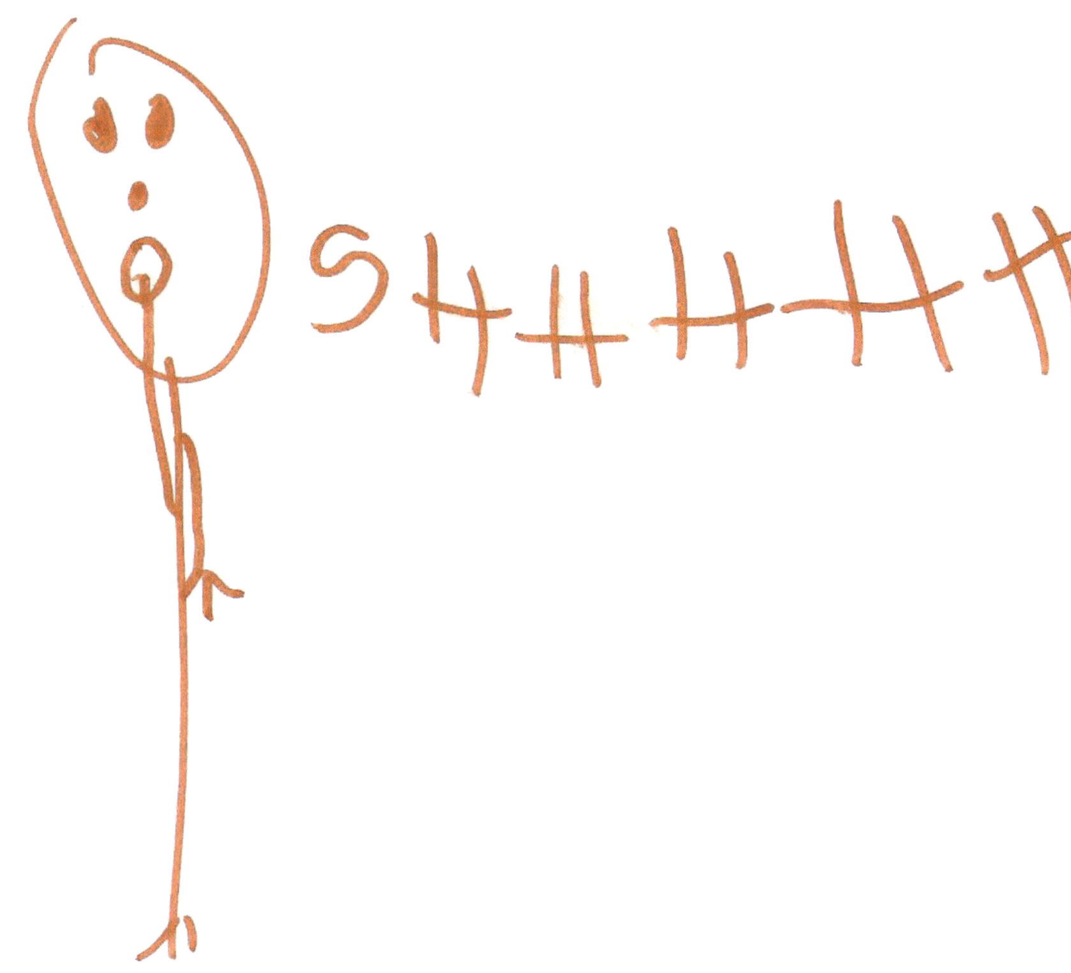

Why did everyone tell her that the baby
was sleeping and that Katie needed to be
quiet?

Katie's mommy gave her a big hug and looked into her big blue eyes.

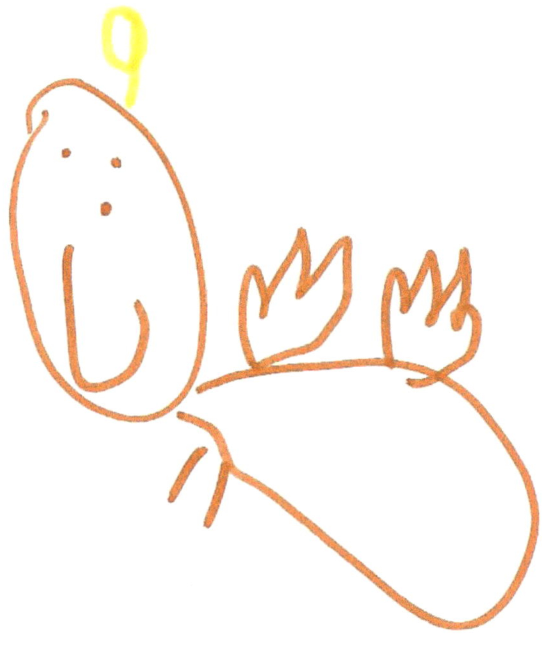

"Do you know what an Angel Baby is?" she asked Katie. Katie shook her head no.

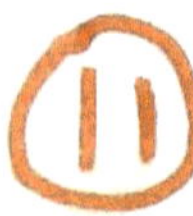

"Sometimes God gives mommies babies in their tummies that come out after a long, long time and stay here on earth. We love that, right?"

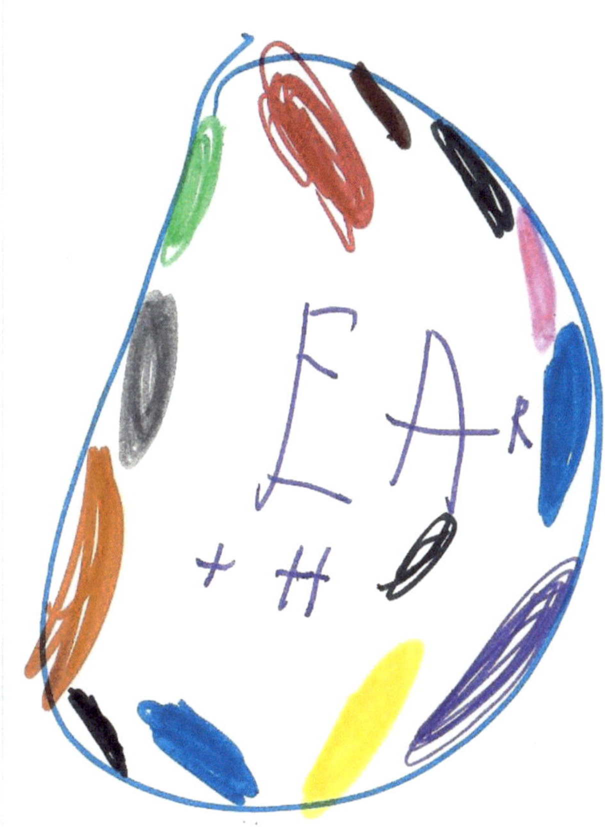

Katie nodded yes.

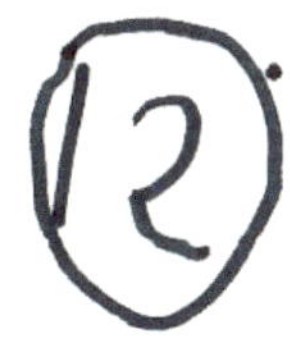

"But sometimes, God gives mommies babies in their tummies that are the most special babies of all … *Angel Babies*."

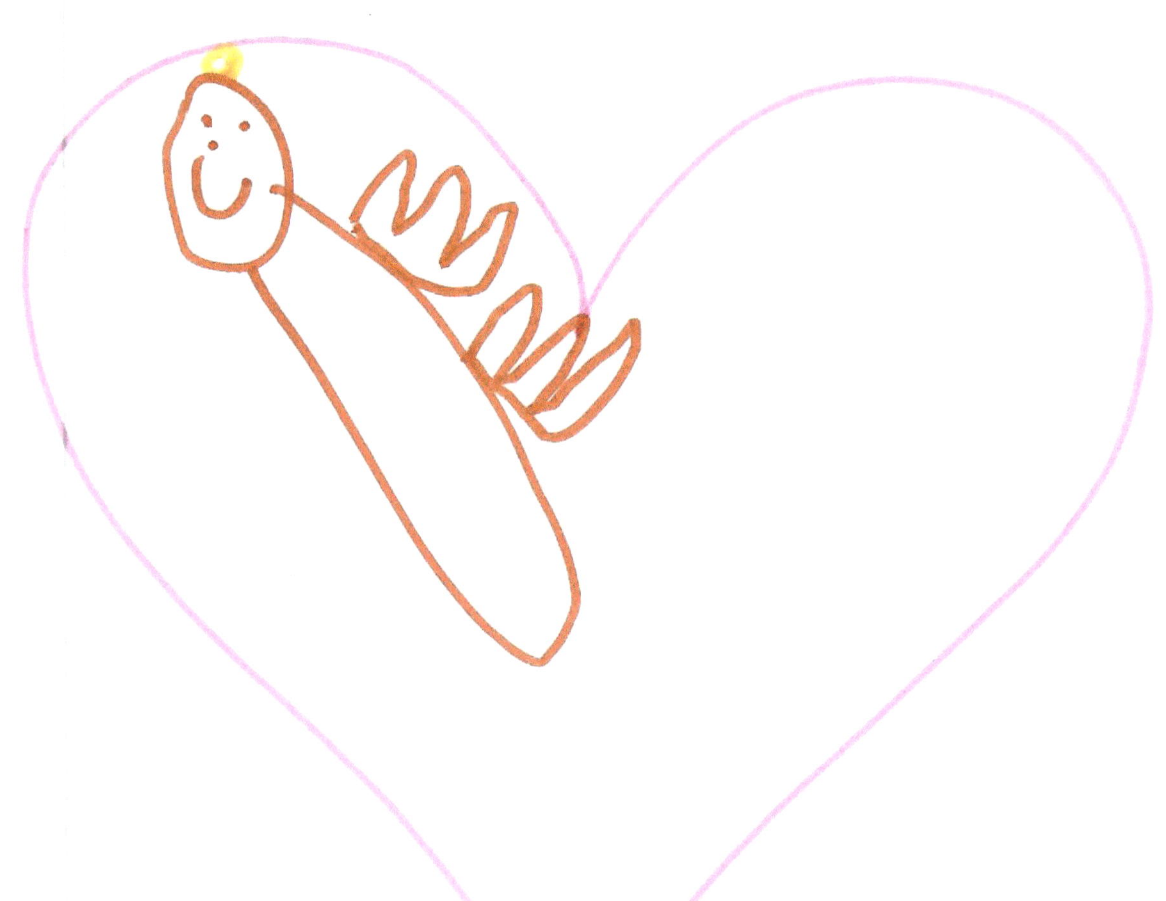

"They grow in our hearts and give us hope. They bring families together."

Katie's mommy made a sad face.

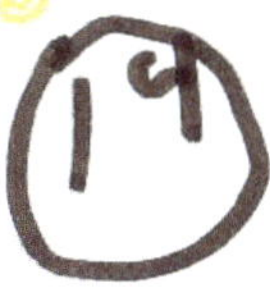

"Now I have to tell you something sad
about Angel Babies."

19

"We don't get to meet Angel Babies here on earth. Before they can be born, they die and go to heaven to be with Jesus."

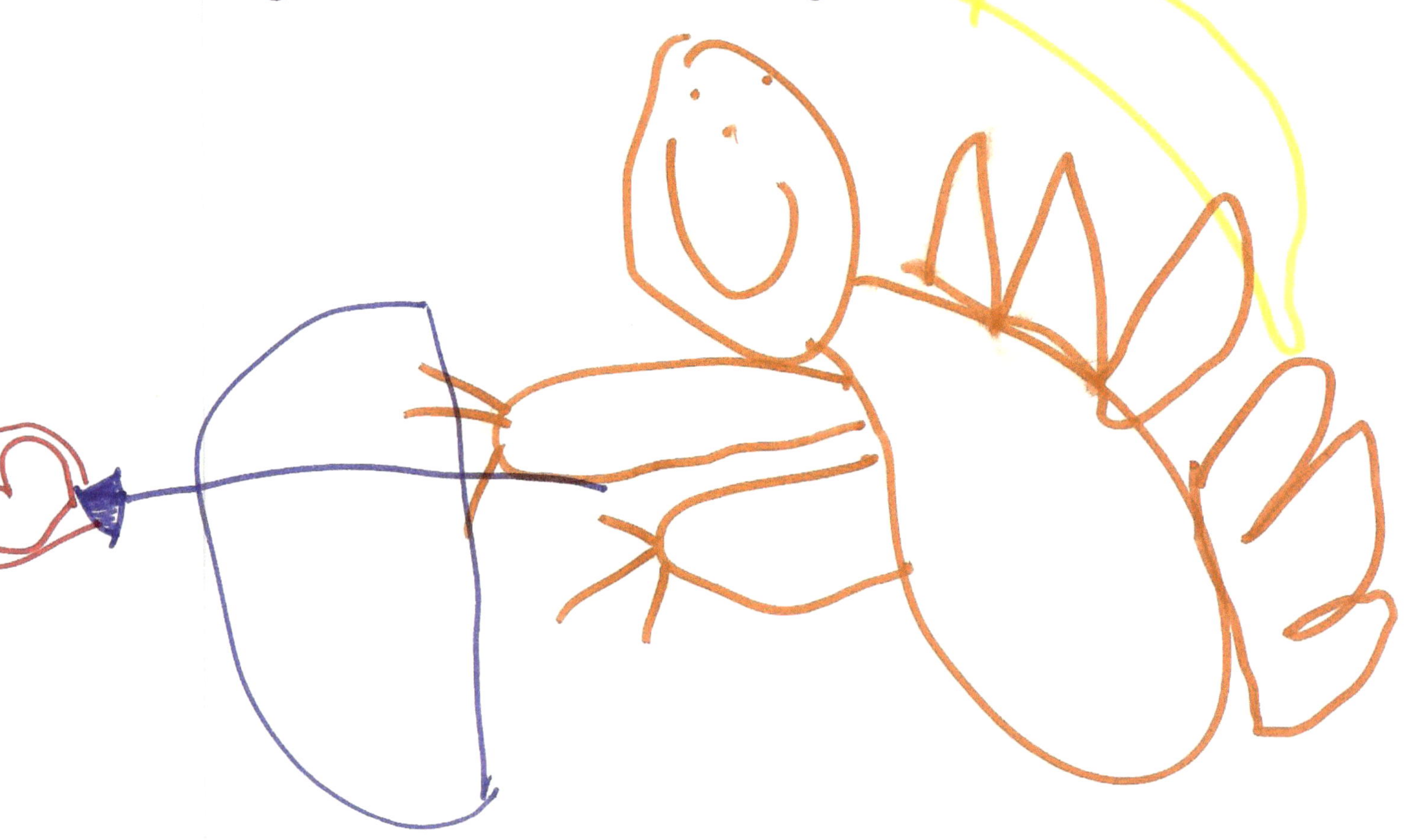

"You see," Katie's mommy continued, "Angel Babies have a very special job ...

"... They prepare us to love all of the babies that He is going to send into our lives in all the years to come..."

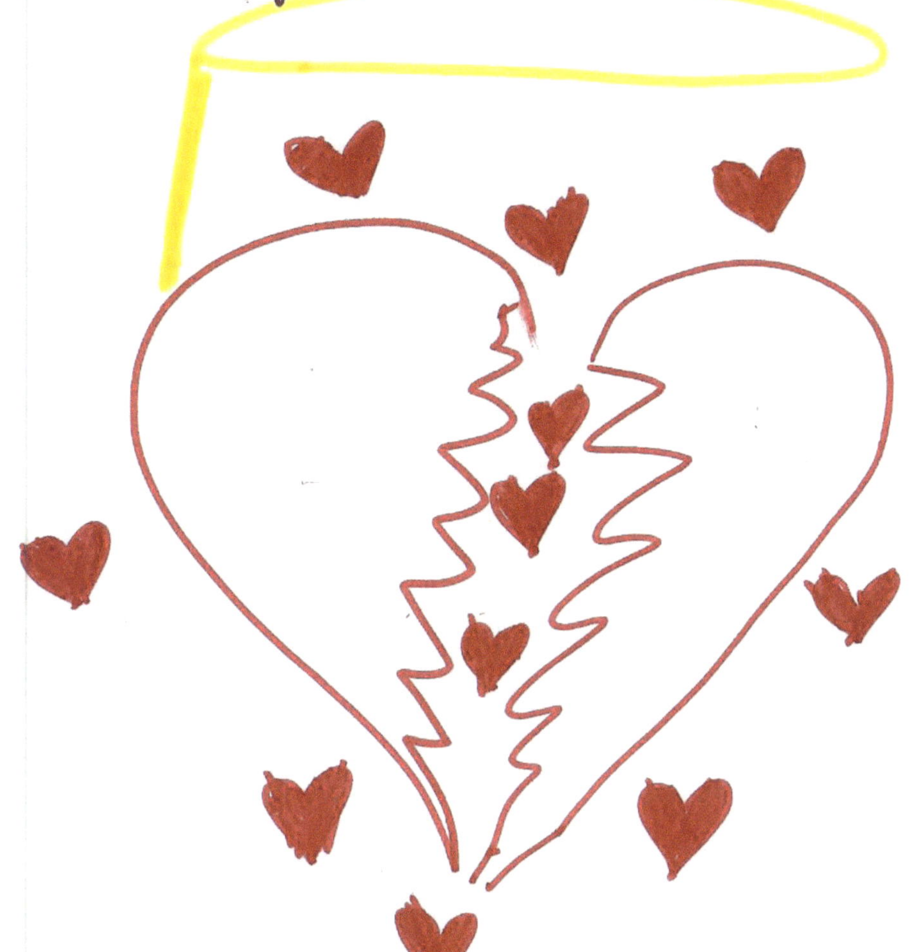

"... And they remind us that the best place to be is heaven, where all of the Angel Babies will be waiting for us, ready to play with them for ever and ever!"

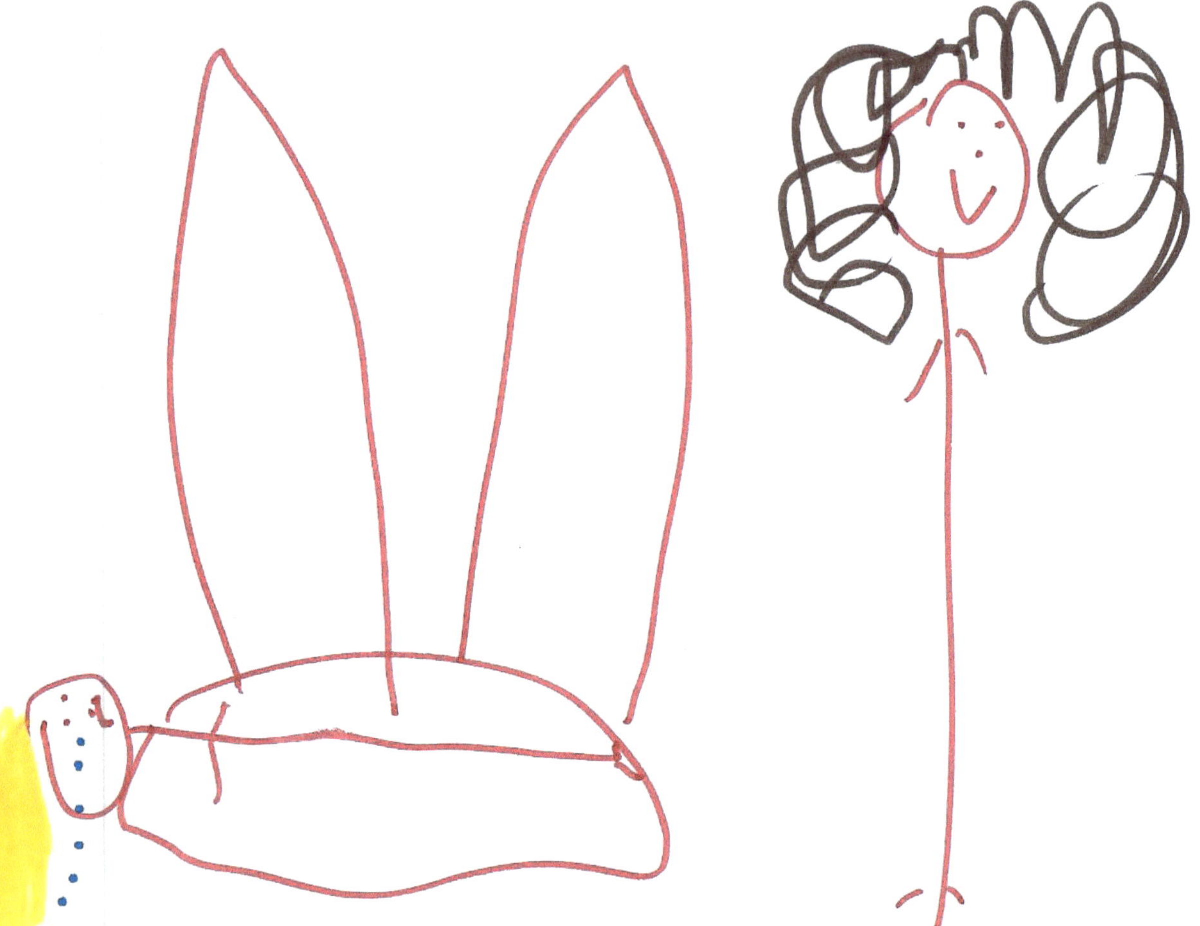

"But if the baby is an Angel Baby and it goes to heaven, then I will miss that baby so much!" Katie cried. "I don't want another baby someday. I love _this_ baby."

17

"We will all miss the baby so much," her mommy said. "That's why your Aunt Jackie is so sad."

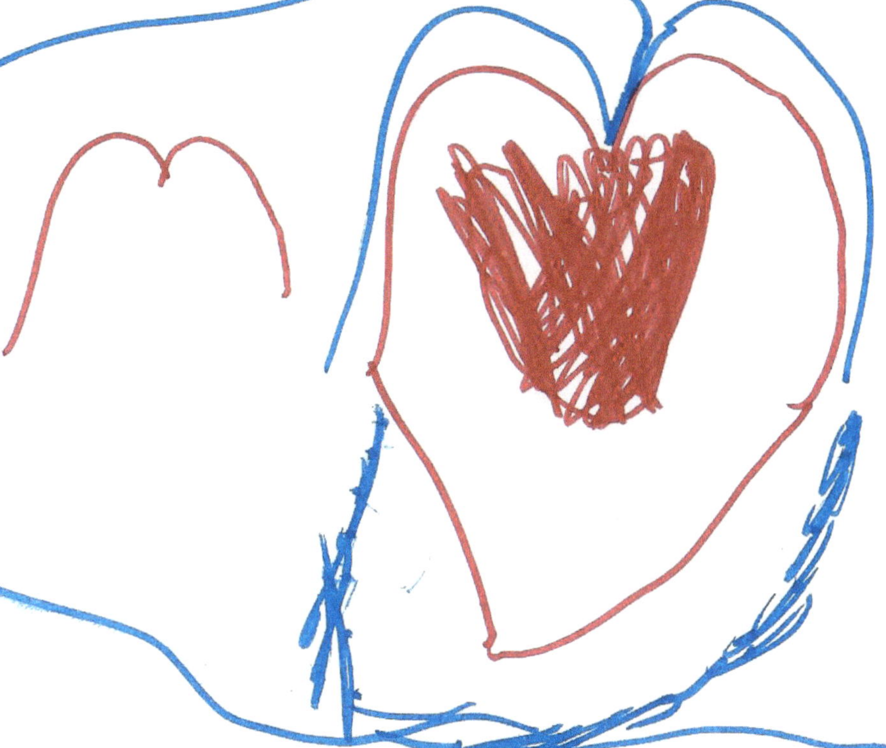

"If her baby is an *Angel Baby*, she will be happy that her baby is going to go straight to heaven, but her heart will be broken because she wanted to keep her baby here with her on earth."

That night, Katie and her mommy prayed
for Aunt Jackie. They prayed that Aunt
Jackie would feel better. They prayed for the
baby in Aunt Jackie's tummy.

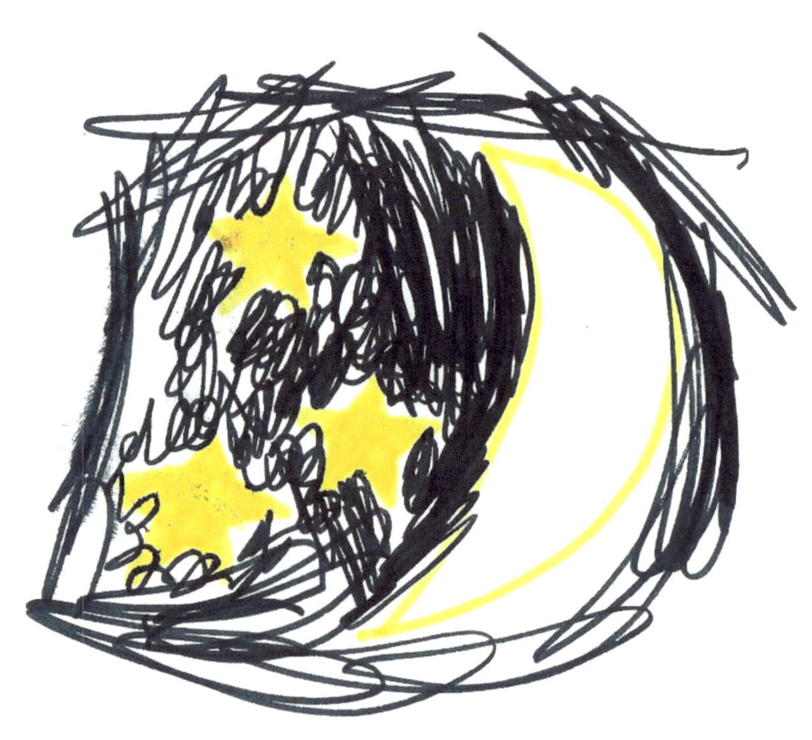

And then, they waited. They waited and
waited to find out if Aunt Jackie's baby was
an Angel Baby or not.

19

The next morning, Katie's Aunt Jackie came over. She told Katie the saddest news ever.

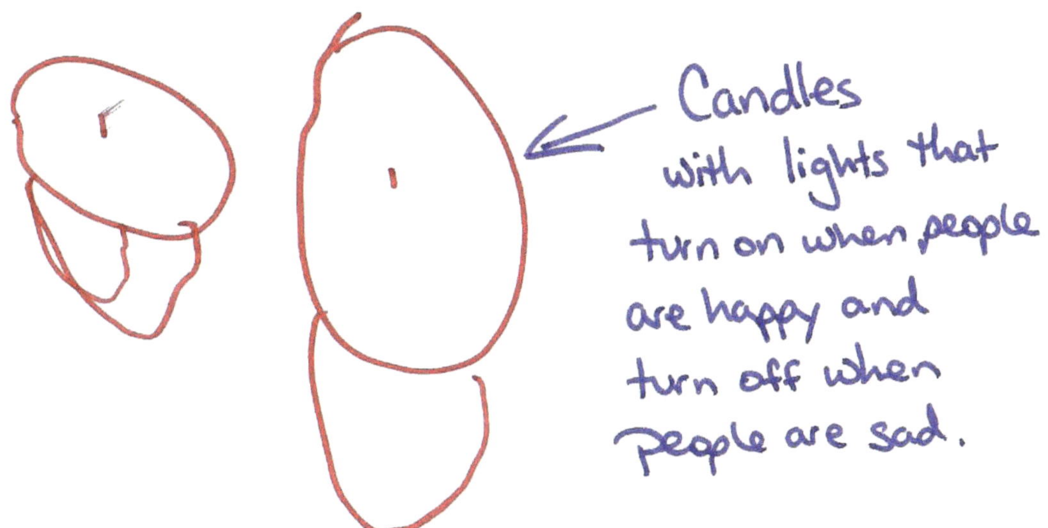

"Katie, my baby isn't in my tummy anymore." Aunt Jackie started to cry.

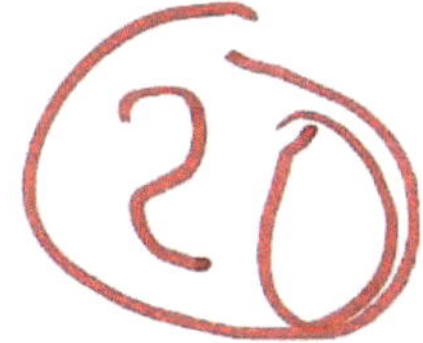

Katie's heart was broken. She had wanted
a new friend to play with here on earth so
badly.

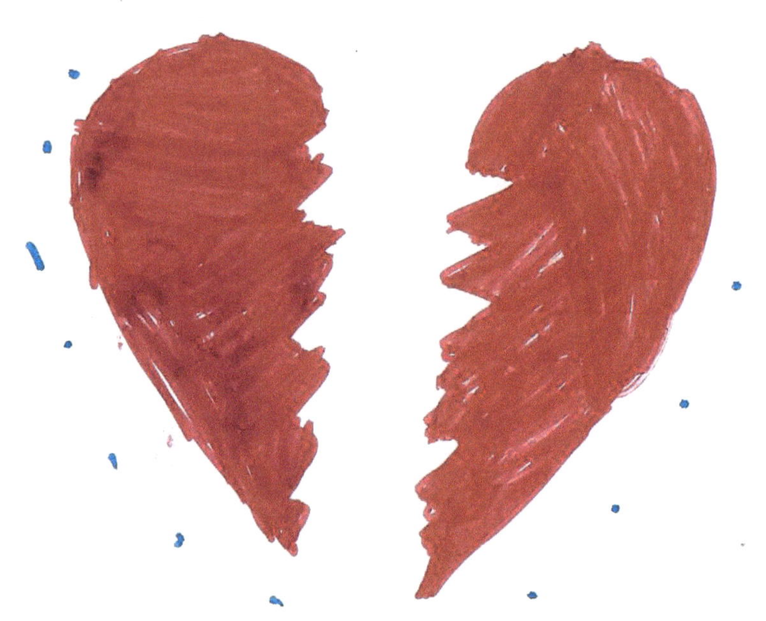

"Don't worry, Aunt Jackie," she sniffed.
"Your baby is in heaven with Jesus! It's an
Angel Baby!"

Katie gave Aunt Jackie the biggest hug ever.

"And because our Angel Baby is in heaven with Jesus, when we go to heaven we can play together! We can have tea parties, and hold the baby, and sing to the baby … forever and ever and ever!"

22

Katie gave a little sigh.

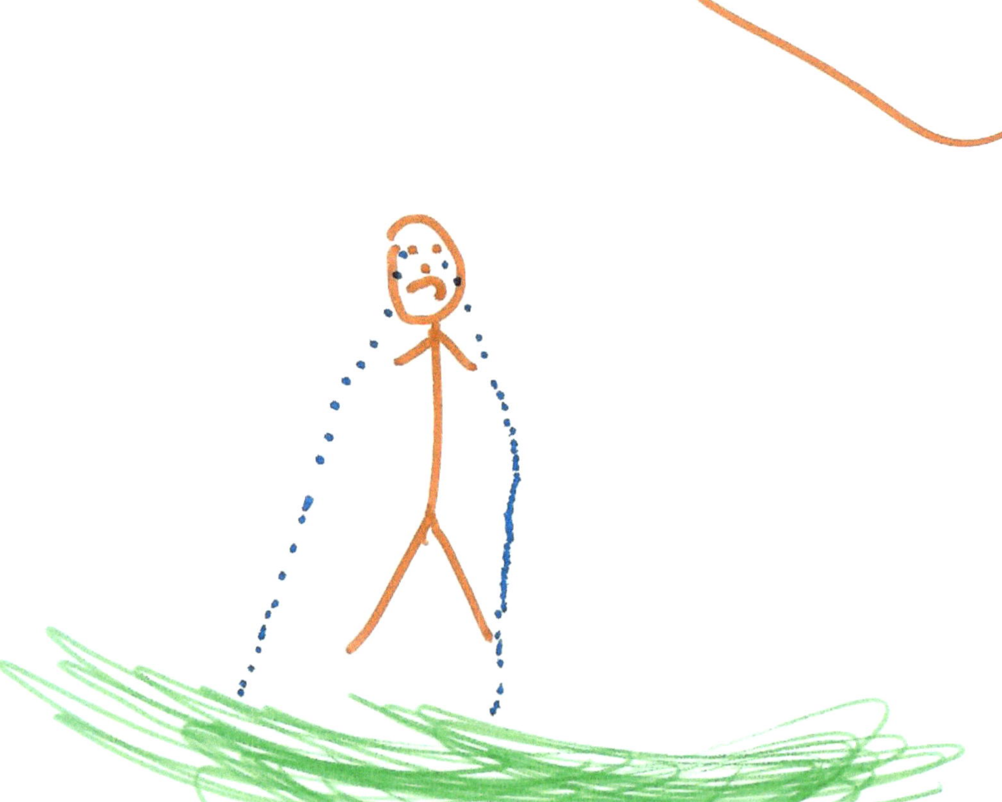

"We'll just have to wait a little longer, that's all."

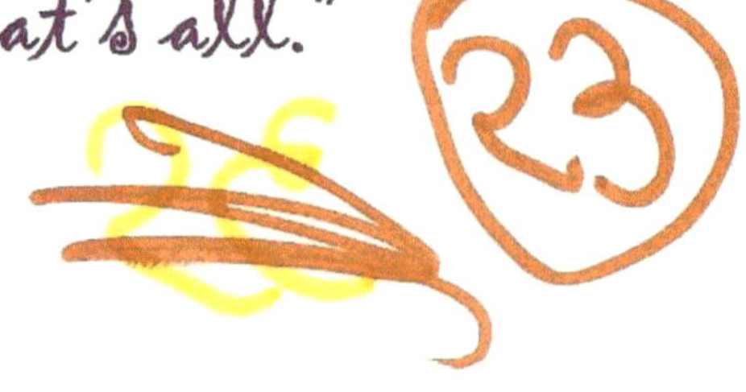

23